BASIC HOME CARE FOR ADVANCED ALS/MND CLIENTS

From a Consumer's Perspective

Okey Nwangburuka, MD

BASIC HOME CARE FOR ADVANCED ALS/MND CLIENTS
Copyright © 2024 by Okey Nwangburuka, MD

ISBN: 979-8895310519 (sc)
ISBN: 979-8895310526 (e)

All rights reserved. No part of this publication may be reproduced, distributed, or transmitted in any form or by any means, including photocopying, recording, or other electronic or mechanical methods, without the prior written permission of the publisher and/or the author, except in the case of brief quotations embodied in critical reviews and other noncommercial uses permitted by copyright law.

The views expressed in this book are solely those of the author and do not necessarily reflect the views of the publisher, and the publisher hereby disclaims any responsibility for them.

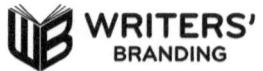

Writers' Branding
(877) 608-6550
www.writersbranding.com
media@writersbranding.com

Contents

WHY THE BOOK? 1

ABOUT THE AUTHOR 3

DEDICATION 5

ACKNOWLEDGEMENTS 7

BIOPSYCHOSOCIAL DIMENSIONS OF THE DISEASE 9

TREATMENTS 10

PREVALENCE AND DIAGNOSTIC PROCEDURES 11

SYMPTOMS MANAGEMENT 11

MORNING ROUTINE 13

CO-MORBID DEPRESSION AND ANXIETY. 15

MORE ON MANAGEMENT OF DEPRESSION /HOPELESSNESS ... 17

MANAGING LOSS OF FINE MOTOR SKILLS 18

MANAGING LOSS OF GROSS MOTOR SKILLS
AND AMBULATION 18

CAREGIVERS 19

MANAGEMENT OF HYPERSECRETIONS 21

MORE ON PERSONAL CARE 21

ABDOMINAL DRESSING 22

CLEANING BOWEL MOVEMENTS 22

MASSAGE 23

BED BATHS	23
MANICURE	24
SUCTION	24
ROOM AIDS	24
THE TRANSFER OF PATIENT TO AND FROM BED TO WHEELCHAIR OR GURNEY!	25
PREPARATION	25
MANAGING RELATIONAL PROBLEMS AND FINANCIAL PLANNING.	27
RECORDING OF CARE, HOME HEALTH VISITS, AND LOCAL RESOURCES	30
CONCLUSION	32
APPENDIX	33
APPENDIX	34

Why the Book?

Amyotrophic Lateral Sclerosis (ALS) is a heterogeneous group of diseases. ALS or "Motor Neuron Disease" as it is called in Britain, or "Maladie de Charcot" in France, is a devastating degenerative illness with no known medical remedy at the time of going to press. Lot of progress has been made in recent years leading to 4 FDA- approved medicines, technological advancements in diagnosis and communication remedies.

The approval of Tofersen for familial ALS associated with the sod1 gene marks a milestone. Research efforts targeting specific immune pathways are ongoing. Other research approaches involving gene-editing, stem cell therapies and targeting specific gene mutations in the field of personalized genetic therapy will hopefully lead the approval of Tofersen for familial ALS associated with sod1 gene marks a milestone. Research efforts targeting specific immune pathways are ongoing.

Other research approaches involve gene-editing, stem cell therapies and targeting specific gene mutations in the field of personalized genetic therapy will hopefully lead to breakthroughs.

Please note that the word 'client' refers to the consumer of health services in any non-hospital setting, whereas 'patient' is associated with hospital services consumers. However, both words are interchangeably used in this mini-book.

At the time the author was diagnosed more than a decade ago, there wasn't enough consumer-centered literature to assist clients and caregivers.

My intention in writing this mini-book is to give both new and more experienced caregivers a quick cheat sheet, when in a fix about what to do for their consumers before professionals are accessed.

Okey Nwangburuka, MD

About the Author

Okey Nwangburuka, MD, was diagnosed with ALS more than a decade ago.

A retired clinical psychiatrist, he had four board certifications before the physical and emotional ravages of the disease forced him into an administrative role in his career.

Dr. Okey lives in California with his children.

Dedication

to

Nonye, Emeka, Eze, Ogechi!

Acknowledgements

With gratitude and humility, I acknowledge the contributions of all doctors, nurses, social workers, janitors, chaplains, OT, PTs , nutritionists, pharmacists, administrative staff, friends, foes, family, intercessors, speech pathologists, research heads and assistants, and others too numerous to mention, I am grateful for what you have taught me, grateful our paths crossed, grateful to you for enriching my life the way you did.

Most especially, to all the caregivers who have helped me be, and continue on this miracle journey. I thank you all.

BIOPSYCHOSOCIAL DIMENSIONS OF THE DISEASE

Amyotrophic Lateral Sclerosis (ALS) is a heterogeneous group of diseases. ALS or "Motor Neuron Disease" as it is called in Britain, or "Maladie de Charcot" in France, is a devastating degenerative illness with no known medical remedy at the time of going to press. However, a company called Neuralinks has successfully completed its first robotic surgery with brain implants to aid paralyzed clients in making movements by thinking of procedure.

A lot of progress has been made in recent years leading to 4 FDA- approved medicines, technological advancements in diagnosis, and communication remedies. The approval of Tofersen for familial ALS associated with the sod1 gene marks a milestone. Research efforts targeting specific immune pathways are, however, ongoing.

Other research approaches involve gene-editing, stem cell therapies, and targeting specific gene mutations in the field of personalized genetic therapy will hopefully lead to breakthroughs.

While some cases of ALS run in families, others are sporadic. Symptoms generally involve the dying of motor neurons throughout the brain, spinal cord, and peripheral nervous systems. These lead to paralysis, loss of speech, and loss of gross and fine motor skills. Total paralysis and pseudobulbar symptoms are fairly common. The prognosis remains abysmal.

This can, however, be improved by giving the client reasons to fight on, holding onto hope, giving back in a non-transactional way, and establishing a link to useful resources, including the medical team. There are interventional studies, observational studies, and historical surveys, as well as voice tracking and other forms of gene studies going on to help find a cure for ALS. It is important to note that frontotemporal dementia is a significant co- morbidity.

Therapeutic resources for caregivers include teaching them caregiver recharge, resilience, and mindful movement. Mindfulness-based therapies, blend Zen, Yoga, and breathing techniques. Through calming of the mind, calmness of the body is achieved!

TREATMENTS

As of the time of going to press, there are 4 approved medicines, as already stated. Neuralinks is working on brain-computer interfaces, activation of brain parts by neural stimulation, and robotic surgery. The medicines prolong life for about six months. Many intolerable side effects make compliance difficult. There are unconventional and unapproved and some dangerous treatments. Always consult with your advanced illness management team before taking to any course of action.

The approval of Tofersen for familial ALS associated with the sod1 gene marks a milestone. Research efforts targeting specific immune pathways are, however, ongoing.

Other research approaches involve gene editing, stem cell therapies, and targeting specific gene mutations in the field of personalized genetic therapy will hopefully lead to breakthroughs.

A bioengineering firm, VentecLife, pioneered a breakthrough by bringing all the bulky equipment required by clients into a piece of portable five-in- one equipment. So, the formerly bulky equipment which has the ventilator, oxygen concentrator, nebulizer, humidifier, and suction machine was simplified into a portable one that's easier for the use of the patient.

Some clients have, however, been hesitant to sign up for use out of fear that if a part malfunctions, repair may involve delays, especially where their distributorships/vendors are still being grown.

PREVALENCE AND DIAGNOSTIC PROCEDURES

The prevalence of ALS in the USA is about 9/100,000 people in the population. Incidence amongst men is slightly higher than in women.

ALS remains a diagnosis of exclusion. Blood, urine, spinal fluid tests, EMG, and NCV studies are all helpful in excluding other illnesses.

SYMPTOMS MANAGEMENT

Symptoms before confirmation of diagnosis of ALS may include fasciculations, spasms, restlessness, fatigability, loss of use of major joints, and non-specific symptoms from every tissue.

After the diagnosis has changed from probable ALS to confirmed ALS, the goal of treatment is to prolong course, minimize complications, manage side effects, and inspire hope while preparing for the eventuality of transition to the other side of eternity.

While still ambulatory, the client may be able to feed with assistance using special cutlery and wear rubberized waist trousers. The occupational therapist will guide the patient in these matters. Change shirts from buttons to Velcro.

Before the total loss of speech, one may use cards if unable to buy anelectronic computerized generating device. If one's occupation involves person-to-person verbal interactions, when the voice becomes quite unintelligible, it's time to quit.

If the body part that is highly involved in the performance of one's career or job becomes heavily affected, it is time to consider quitting.

A disability van and wheelchair with a ramp for access will be necessary. The local ALS Association can assist in directing one to secure an affordable car for purchase or lease when needed. Most importantly, peer support groups and family support are very important.

Bulking up weight in anticipation of muscle loss and atrophy becomes indicated i f the nutritionist or MD advises. I found H2cal particularly helpful. Some of the side effects, however, include constipation and ease of fullness. Adding fiber and using stool softeners may be helpful.

It is important to know when to cut back on work and when to stop work! Once a diagnosis is confirmed, the patient/client will be fast-tracked onto Medicare. One must be aware that Medicare requires an annual report of how your disability checks are spent if any savings are made. If you have an appointed representative, they can help with the report.

Unfortunately, a time comes when the swallowing ability becomes highly compromised. Within the progression from solid to liquid food, the need for a gastro-jejunal tube will arise.

By this time, all peripheral muscles except the sex organ and to a lesser extent, eye muscles are unaffected. When this happens, almost all balance is lost and the client becomes quadriplegic!

Let's switch gears to taking care of the quadriplegic ALS patient.

MORNING ROUTINE

This refers to the processes for getting the client ready in the morning upon awakening. These processes you will find repeated through other parts of day and night. So, if new caregivers are being trained, morning hours may be the most conducive for that.

- With a warm towel, wipe the face.
- Suction mouth and nose

If necessary, do a deep suction, to relieve chest congestion. In the event of dry eyes, give eye drops.

Reposition parts of the body such as legs, palms, elbows, and head. Give oral care! Chlorhexidine is often prescribed.

Because patients with respiratory organ failure are intubated while hospitalized, their dentition aesthetics may be negatively impacted.

Having a dental hygienist visit at home monthly or quarterly may be useful.

Regular ENT and GP/PCP visits a n d pulmonologists cannot be over-emphasized.

Do neck dressing daily and change the inner cannula every other day.

The Portex or other brand of tracheostomy instrument is changed in an ENT doctor's office every six to eight weeks.

Moving and transporting the patient from his bed is usually cumbersome for the client. Pain, anxiety, and breathing problems are worsened. **Caregivers with experience devise their methods to make the burden lighter on the patient.**

G-tube dressing: should be done daily. Tape it close to the G-tube to hold it in place. If the G- tube comes off, call 911 or your interventional radiology department.,

Cleaning bowel movements: Done on patient patient-required basis, plus every morning.

Body wash: Done at least once daily.

Feeding: This should be according to the doctor's or nutritionist's recommendation. There are various formulae commercially available.

Medications: Should be administered as per doctor's orders via the g-tube.

Cover the client's body according to personal preferences. Be aware that being very hot could trigger chest congestion and respiratory distress.

MANAGEMENT OF WEIGHT LOSS

- Anticipate weight loss even before a diagnosis is confirmed.

- This is the time to increase weight healthily before weight loss ensues.

- Bulk up, there are high-calorie formulas commercially available. An example is H2cal.

- Balance the above supplements or main food with fruits and vegetables.

- Monitor and treat changes in bowel movements. Also, include fiber if tolerated.

- Monitor and report weight regularly to health care providers and nutritionists.

CO-MORBID DEPRESSION AND ANXIETY.

Treatment of the above should be part of a client's tailored comprehensive treatment plan. Non-pharmacological and pharmacological approaches are both effective.

Pharmacological approaches include the use of SSRIs and SNRIs.

Sometimes short-term benzodiazepines, beta-blockers, mood-stabilizing agents, or typical anti-psychotics can be added to enhance efficacy.

Monitor for side effects, especially for suicidal ideations or self-injurious impulses. Sometimes some clients are allowed to continue on medications longer than usual to improve quality of life in a "terminal" condition.

Non-pharmacological approaches include cognitive behavioral therapy, interpersonal therapy, and problem-solving therapies.

Good sleep hygiene, addressing dietary issues, the practice of meditation, yoga as applicable, and other mindfulness-based techniques can be effective.

Addressing pain issues is also necessary. Often, clients may not tolerate some techniques which is why treatment is tailored to individual needs.

Needless to say, because of paralysis, yoga is not positional in nature.

The home health nurse can follow up on checking on progress and side effects in between visits with therapists or physicians.

MORE ON MANAGING FEAR AND ANXIETY.

- Anxiety and related fears of dying, and leaving loved ones behind can be pervasive and all-consuming, especially after diagnosis is probable or confirmed.

- The intensity varies depending on the age of diagnosis, sense of accomplishment in life, support systems, access to health care, and finances.

- Untreated anxiety makes the prognosis worse.

- Support groups, contingency management, and individual therapy are helpful.

- If necessary, consult with a health care provider about anti-anxiety medication.

MORE ON MANAGEMENT OF DEPRESSION / HOPELESSNESS

- Significant symptoms of depression within the context of a severe medical illness include anhedonia, hopelessness, and suicidal or self-harm ideations.

- Adaptive sadness is normal.

- Support of loved ones, allowing for space to mourn loss once in a while is helpful!

- Individual, and group therapies, and spiritual reflections with a chaplain are also necessary.

- If antidepressants are necessary, give it a trial.

- There's more to life, even after the loss of functions. Having supportive, positively-minded caregivers is key to environmental management.

Caregivers should be encouraging but not give false hope. However, do not give up on hope. Do not dwell on the past. Faith-based therapies and rituals such as prayers, chants, songs, worshiping, holy communion, anointing with oil, fasting, etc. may be beneficial.

MANAGING LOSS OF FINE MOTOR SKILLS

This occurs early with disease onset. Working with your occupational therapist helps incredibly with ways and devices to assist with clothing, handwriting, use of cutlery, etc. Appropriate use of over-the-counter joint- holding equipment is helpful.

The treatment team is best constituted if your visits include sessions with RN, OT, PT, and speech pathologist, all on the same day.

MANAGING LOSS OF GROSS MOTOR SKILLS AND AMBULATION

When gross motor skills gradually decline, ambulation, neck-holding, and inability to function without help can be overwhelming for the family and caregivers.

The living space often does require accommodations. Ramps, wide-enough hallways, bathroom renovations with shower/bath accommodations. Eventually, all of these will not be conducive, when total paralysis sets in. Bed baths are done daily or as tolerated.

Room aeration and aromatization may be useful if clients have frequent visitors. Strollers, manual wheelchairs, motorized wheelchairs, and disability vehicles are often necessary.

The skills of transferring from bed to ambulatory aid, or disability vehicle require some clinical training.

For the transfer to and from the bed, motorized or manual lifts are employed. Hoyer Lifts is a popular commercial brand. Caregivers must ensure motorized equipment is charged.

If a client is on a permanent vent, please ensure there is a backup, and do keep it charged always.

Mechanical ventilators should also be handy. In the event of power failure, there should be a standby generator! I f the city utilities department has the resources, clients should be enlisted for medical disability services.

CAREGIVERS

This section will focus on qualities desirable in caregivers.

It is fairly easy to present well and say the right things during an interview. A two-week training period can serve as an extended interview.

Empathy, giving care with mindfulness of clients' dignity, long-suffering, and humility are better observed than talked about.

Caregivers should also be treated with responsiveness, respect, and grace, realizing mistakes are made sometimes.

The ability to be calm under emergency circumstances is vital. Willingness to keep improving as opposed to arrogance and a haughty attitude are vital.

Caregivers should cross-train on every aspect of the job; routine activities, wheelchair ambulation, companionship, accompaniment to clinic, emergency room visits, and present if hospitalization occurs.

House cleaning chores may be necessary depending on the home circumstances.

These requirements should be made clear as part of the job description.

Helping clients take calls or make calls, texts, and emails should be minimized for clients' sense of privacy. This is not always possible as it requires additional financial resources.

A non - in - depth education about the unconscious motivations that influence our quality of relationships and reactions to clients will help caregivers be more psychologically aware.

Bringing the unconscious into the conscious realm will improve their quality of care and their interpersonal relationships significantly.

Once or twice yearly meet and greet by the advanced illness management group nurse can be the venue for this.

It is important to encourage caregivers to attend local ALS association meetings from time to time, to be part of the community, build resilience, and refresh their knowledge base. Helping caregivers build resilience reduces attrition from burnout.

MANAGEMENT OF HYPERSECRETIONS

In light of the respiratory failure that accompanies this stage of disease, hypersecretions can present a challenging source of regular discomfort. Medications, patches, and frequent suctioning are necessary. Often the employment of medicines and patches can lead to bronchial mucus plugs.

As stated earlier, bronchial washout in a hospital setting may be needed if breathing becomes severely impeded.

Regular oral, nasal, and chest (deep) suctioning will reduce discomfort. For clients living at home, caregivers can do all of these.

Respiratory therapists can train caregivers. The use of wet towels will prevent skin dryness. The use of lip balms will help prevent lip dryness.

MORE ON PERSONAL CARE

The morning routine involves most of the training curricula except processes such as inventory, equipment management, and house chores.

Typically, before a client is discharged to the home, an assigned caregiver is trained by a respiratory therapist or a home health nurse.

The trained caregiver can then train others. Let's review some "morning routine" procedures Neck dressing Bring out a pre-arranged pack and open it. Spread out utensils to use.

With gauze, clean around the trachea wound.

Using a Q-tip in a pack, try to remove dirty blood particles. Dry with new gauze.

Place completely new gauze after applying anti-itch cream.

Tie velcro belt. Using two fingers, run across the velcro belt to ensure it is not too tight.

Abdominal Dressing

- Do not overexpose the body.

- Hold the g-tube down, and clean around with gauze and a Q-tip.

- Do not try to clean "one hundred percent" because the wound is fresh.

- Apply fresh gauze in opposite directions.

- Using medical tape, band closer to the entry point of the tube in four directions.

- Close the body with sheets.

Cleaning bowel movements

Each caregiver eventually adopts a method best suited for them. Ensure the patient is well-cleaned before changing pads.

Massage

Frequent massaging with skillful hands or massage guns relieves pain and improves circulation.

Personal grooming such as haircuts, styling, pedicures, and manicures should not be forgotten in the hustle and bustle of care management. When necessary, be guided by a licensed professional.

Range of motion exercises, as tolerated, help reduce stiffness and flaccidity in earlier phases of illness.

Again, we are dealing with clients with advanced-stage illness, but in the beginning, muscle relaxants, prednisone, can reduce muscle spasms, and fasciculations.

When in advanced stages of illness, if a client chooses not to go with hospice care, mild to moderate doses of morphine can be very helpful. Additionally, a very small dose of Benzo can take the edge off pain and morbid anxiety.

Bed baths

Bed baths and toileting were discussed in the early chapter. A bed bath involves the appropriate cleaning of a totally paralyzed client without the added stress of putting on a wheelchair to give a shower in the family bathroom.

- Add moisturizer and Dettol antiseptic to water of desired temperature.

- Using face towels to wipe down.
- Dry each part of the body sectionally.
- When done, moisturize if requested by the client.

Remember patient's breathing is compromised when laid flat below thirty degrees for a significant length of time.

Manicure

- When a manicure or pedicure is being done, be careful not to induce whitlow infections or cut/brush too deep.
- Watch for pressure sores and bedsores. Prevention is better here, remember.
- In the event of pressure sores, report to PCP immediately.
- Change position on a bed frequently. Some hospital beds can be bought for home use and provide this preventive function!

Suction

It is important to suction off fluid accumulating in the lungs. Sometimes regular chest or deep suction is not enough. There is equipment that is designed for chest vibrations. Some can be used at home. Others are only used in hospital settings by respiratory therapists.

Room Aids

Fortunately, there are smart aids such as Google Smart Hub and Alexa that can help clients control TVs, air conditioners, heaters, home curtains, and front door, visitors. These tech aids can help clients stay in touch with parts of their homes.

No recording aid should be installed in bedrooms, bathrooms, or otherwise private parts of the home because that is illegal in most states.

Keeping the client intellectually or spiritually stimulated is a healthy distraction from the ever-ubiquitous noise of impending doom.

Another important technological aid is the speech-generating device. There are open- source SGDs on the market but the Tobii-dynavox seems to be recommended by most speech pathologists.

With this, clients can communicate by voice, text, and email, and remain active on social media platforms. The frustration of prolonged silence can be a killer and worsen prognosis.

THE TRANSFER OF PATIENT TO AND FROM BED TO WHEELCHAIR OR GURNEY!

Transferring a paralyzed patient on a ventilator from a bed to a wheelchair requires careful planning and execution to ensure the safety and comfort of the patient. Here is a general outline of the process:

Preparation

– Ensure the patient's ventilator is portable or has sufficient battery charge for the duration of the transfer.

- Prepare the wheelchair, adjusting the seat, footrests, and other supports.

- Gather necessary equipment like a transfer board, slide sheet, or mechanical lift, depending on the patient's needs and capabilities.

- Check the patient's medical devices (e.g., ventilator tubes, IV lines, catheters) to ensure they are secure and won't be dislodged during the transfer.

- Ensure that the bed is locked and stable.

- Explain the process to the patient, if they are conscious, to help reduce anxiety and ensure cooperation.

- Position the patient close to the edge of the bed on their side facing the wheelchair.

- Use a transfer board or slide sheet under the patient to facilitate a smooth transfer.

- With one or more caregivers, use the chosen transfer method (manual, slide sheet, transfer board, mechanical or electronic lift) to move the patient from the bed to the wheelchair.

Ensure that the patient's ventilator and other medical equipment move with the patient and remain functional.

- Position the patient comfortably in the wheelchair, ensuring they are properly supported.

- Secure any safety belts or restraints.

- Adjust the ventilator and any other medical equipment.
- Check the patient for any discomfort or issues following the transfer.
- Ensure the patient is well-positioned, with the ventilator and other devices properly set up.

It's crucial to have trained healthcare professionals conduct or supervise this transfer, as the process requires specific skills and knowledge, particularly in handling a ventilator- dependent patient.

It's important to remember to plug in the ventilator to recharge, reconnect the oxygen tube, and reset the speech-generating device, phone, and suction machine in previously set parameters.

The transfer from the bed allows for changing of the bed-sheets and scrubbing down the mattress with antiseptic.

MANAGING RELATIONAL PROBLEMS AND FINANCIAL PLANNING.

The diagnosis of ALS may sound insurmountable but it is also an opportunity to keep one's house in order. Try to make peace with friends and foes, ask for, and give forgiveness, practice prayers and alms giving, etc.

You will find that many you thought were friends were not really friends. Some stay for a season, some stay for a period, but only those who stay till the end with you truly care for you. But this is no time for grudges, bitterness or unforgiveness. There is a bigger picture to focus on. Fighting off the impossible. Hoping against hope so you can live as fully as you can. It is also the time to put your financial house in order as well.

A last testament and will, an estate planning trust, where applicable, the appointment of a medical and general DPOA (durable power of attorney), and reassuring your close loved ones of your love as frequently as possible.

As much as we are encouraged to hope against hope, believing that with God, all things are possible, it could also end up gloriously with clients going to meet their maker.

The DPOA doesn't have to be family or a friend. Some professionals do it for a fee.

If you are single and never made a move to communicate your feelings to the other, this is a good time to fulfill your dreams.

Do not let the disease stop you from fulfilling your destiny. Any uncompleted project should be completed. The expectation of a better tomorrow is often self-fulfilling. Live life to the fullest every day. It is not easy to do some of the things suggested above.

Permit me please to share a short, edited excerpt on forgiveness from my book **"A-B-C's SUCCESS FOR THE TEEN SOUL, VOLUME ONE"**.

That which I behold I will eventually hold! Forgiveness is forgiving and not withholding.

That which I help release to others will be returned to me.

I will forgive even as I am forgiven. I will not be ruled by my emotions but I must pay attention to what my emotions are trying to tell me about me.

This is an expensive gift that you may not be ready to give because the pain cuts deep when the offense is perpetrated by close loved ones!

Offenses, conflicts, and disputes do occur in life! Even abuses and conscious or unconscious hurting of each other. They do because we are not perfect!

I have blind spots, personality differences, and different life experiences from others.

Even open, honest, self-disclosing, and radically transparent communication do not prevent conflicts.

I must therefore be open to the concept of thoughtful disagreements and useful chaos! My feelings come and go.

Even my thoughts and beliefs evolve, But I will walk in my current illumination while seeking more enlightenment.

Relinquishing all preconceived notions in search of the truth that liberates! My apologies will be authentic, from my heart, and without pretentiousness. I will be quick to say I am sorry and ask for forgiveness when appropriate. I will forgive so I can heal. An act of self-love!

I will learn all that I need to learn from the situation or conflict that gave rise to the need for forgiveness.

I will gladly receive the forgiveness offered to me, both vertically and horizontally, and never take it for granted!

I choose to be joyful, thankful, hopeful, and forgiving today. I don't fully understand it but there seems to be a thread that links these to facing life's challenges better!

I choose to be joyfully expectant of good things. I have hope! I offer respect and recognize the God-given dignity in all others! I will not cease to wonder, be curious, or live amazed.

When down and difficult times come, I pray and meditate for patience! Patience to be still and know that this too will pass. I will recognize and imbibe consciously the power of hope, thanksgiving, and forgiveness.

I will forgive even in circumstances I cannot change, and situations that defer hope. Forgiveness gives me victory, not as much as it does to the one I am giving it to.

- Help the client to live in greater consciousness of the love and favor of God than in the fear of the burden of a beaten beast.

- Give the client opportunities to laugh e.g., by watching comedies, reminiscing on happy times, use of imagery. "A merry heart doeth good like medicine". Laughter remains good medicine.

RECORDING OF CARE, HOME HEALTH VISITS, AND LOCAL RESOURCES.

Granted that this mini-book focuses on the care of the advanced ALS client in the home setting, an effort should be made to record the care given.

- Record times and doses of medications given.

- Record the volume of food consumed and time given.

- Record side effects of medication, duration, and symptoms.

- Write down vitals, weight, and estimated pain (zero to ten).

- You may request weight measurement in the hospital whenever the client visits there.

- Estimation of pain is subjective, please record at least thrice weekly.

- BP, temperature, pulse ox, and heart rate, can be measured by using an affordable smartwatch. An example is smartwatch from smartwatch12 dot com.

Usually, if a client refuses hospice care, he is assigned to an advanced illness management team headed often by a home health nurse who will visit weekly or biweekly until discharge from visitations. Follow-up afterward is by phone. The team must be kept up to date about the client's symptoms, signs, progress, or otherwise!

- Your neurology/ALS team including RT, OT, PT, Specialist Nurses, and Speech therapist.

- Your advanced illness management team.

- Your chaplain.

- Your loved ones, and family.

- Your local ALS association.

The role of local ALS associations cannot be overemphasized. They provide equipment on loan and connect you to resources for paying for services or procuring disability vehicles. They offer care support training, caregiver community activities, professional seminars on ALS, and advocacy efforts for those affected by ALS.

– Your primary care provider.

These are your important clinical resources. Persons of faith have in addition pastors, prophets, and intercessors. It is rare unless personally paid for to have an individual therapist at advanced stages of illness.

CONCLUSION

Again, to re-emphasize, the diagnosis strikes fear. It is still considered incurable. But do not give up without a fight. Fight, for your loved ones, to fulfill your destiny, and to glorify your higher power. If you don't give in and give up, hopefully together with your support, what seems to be the end of the road will turn out to be just a bend, or a T-junction.

APPENDIX

Pictures of some equipment

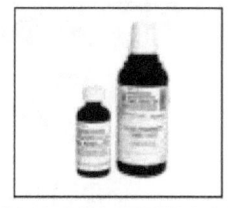
CHLORHEXIDINE

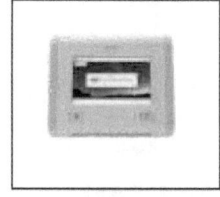
VENTILATOR

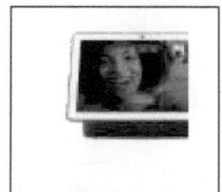
GOOGLE SMART SPEAKER

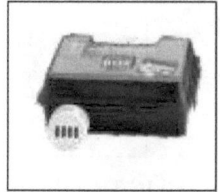
CONTROLLED MEDICATION BOX

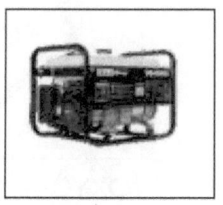
HOME GENERATING SET

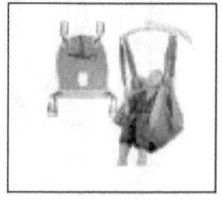
HOYER MAT

APPENDIX

Pictures of some equipment

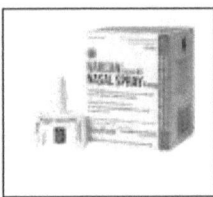
NARCAN NASAL SPRAY

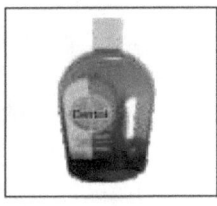
DETTOL

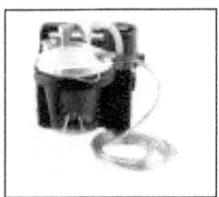
SUCTION MACHINE

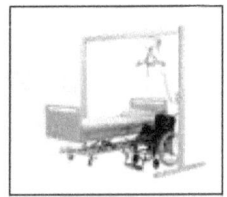
MOLIFTS

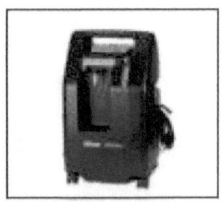
OXYGEN CONCENTRATOR

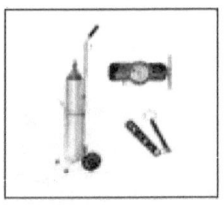
OXYGEN TANK

www.ingramcontent.com/pod-product-compliance
Lightning Source LLC
LaVergne TN
LVHW041600070526
838199LV00046B/2074